24 Energies for Multidimensional Healing

Sara Florida PhD

Copyright © 2017 Sara Florida

All rights reserved.
ISBN: 1545576238
ISBN 13: 9781545576236
Library of Congress Control Number: 2017908141
www.24energies.com
24 Energies for Multidimensional Healing:
Houston, Texas

DEDICATION

This book is an inspiration from my grandfather, who came to me in a dream state vision in which I saw the energies, after he passed to the other side. He was an accomplished scientist during his life, who worked with solar energy and aerospace engineering.

I have been using many of the energies in my healing practice since 2012, and the effects are profound. I have received further visions, showing me that these energies would be beneficial to others for healing at a high vibration.

CONTENTS

Acknowledgments	P 1
Chapter 1: About the Energies, Tachyon & Kryon	P 11
Chapter 2: Preparation and Self-Care for Use	P 14
Chapter 3: Healer Energy Activations	P 28
Chapter 4: How to Invoke the Energies	P 33
Chapter 5: Physical and Emotional Healing Energies	P 41
Chapter 6: Clearing Space and Energy	P 51
Chapter 7: Investigative Energies – Get Answers	P 59
Chapter 8: Vibration-Raising Energies - Consciousness	P 73
Chapter 9: Creation Energies for Manifestation	P 83
Chapter 10: Twin Rays Balancing	P 97
About the Author	P 102
References	P 104

ACKNOWLEDGMENTS

I would like to thank all who have helped me to come to the point where I am now in my sojourn. I have had many teachers, all of whom I give great gratitude. Many of them have been authors and speakers. I have read hundreds of books and attended many healing conferences on self-discovery, healing and spirituality, to reach this point. I would specifically like to thank my grandfather for sharing the energies with me in a vision; Jennifer Buergermeister, who is a mentor for my growth through the practice of yoga and Eastern philosophy; Bing You, MD (China), who is my teacher and mentor in integrated medicine, qigong and tai qi; James Tyberonn of Earth-keepers, who provides life-changing conferences that provide connections and knowledge in earth vortices and specifically training in the Metatronic Keys; Lois Wetzel, who provided spiritual healing and introduced me to higher dimensional healing modalities, Cris Jacinto who gave me the nudge to complete this book, Christopher Morphis for his insight and beautiful art for the cover, as well as Leon Van Kraayenburg for his sacred geometry artwork in the book. The list could go on and on, so I would simply like to send gratitude and love to all those teachers, authors, friends, and family who have played a positive and supportive role in my journey.

Endorsements

" I have been working with these energies for several years with my patients. I am grateful for their help in balancing energy, clearing negative emotions and physical pain. The results are often instantaneous. Thank you Sara for sharing them with me.

~Erika – Houston, TX

"Sara sees beyond. I remember the first time she called in Kryon and Tachyon energies during my healing session. It was as if the whole room filled up with love, and the invocation of the energy invited to help me heal faster and on a deeper level. I've broken barriers with Sara, that no longer took me lifetimes to heal."

~ Katrice G, Houston, TX

"Sara and I became acquainted through her metaphysical group, and we were drawn closer over the years, sharing multidimensional experiences together, making us spiritual sisters. One of these amazing experiences was the birth of her son. We do meditation, energy work, and /or exchanges more consistently with our family and friends. I thoroughly enjoy Sara's work. I used to see her every week and have seen many ailments or concerns go away. It was a pleasure getting a boost and being submerged in loving clarity."

~ Phire, Houston, TX

1 ABOUT THE ENERGIES

The 24 energies are best suited for the healers, who have experience working with energy healing and balancing. These energies work inter-dimensionally. There is a basic assumption that those reading the book have received the necessary training to prepare them for this book. There are many references available, to assist with any areas that the reader may require more study.

These energies are gifts from the divine and are to be cherished by each person who uses hem. These energies are a portion of the key to the higher dimensions. The ability to use these energies opened up and became available fully to humanity in 2012 when the mass consciousness of humanity reached a vibration capable of receiving and using them on a large scale. There are people that have been working with certain forms of the energies for quite some time. The information contained in this book is by no means meant to replace or counter information provided by others for similar work, only to add to or enhance what already exists.

Basis of Tachyon and Kryon Energies

Tachyon healing energy is an energy that has been used by others on this planet for planetary and individual healing and is the basis for some of the energies in the book. Tachyon is the the first energy we discuss will go into more detail in Chapter five Healing Energies. It is an energy that vibrates faster than the speed of light and is self- balancing. According to Dr. Joseph McNamara of Tachyon Counseling, a world leader in tachyon technology information, "Tachyons are subatomic particles that travel faster than light. They are particles that infuse physical matter with spiritual light. Tachyonization is a technological process that impregnates the physical matter with an increased quantity of tachyons and thus it permanently changes quantum properties of atomic nuclei which compose that matter." The energies are received from higher-dimensional realms. They work within the light sphere that surrounds the earth, where human consciousness resides. The earth resonance is ever increasing and vibrating faster as the consciousness of humanity is increasing. As humanity progresses and increases in vibration, our heartbeat is aligning with that of Earth and God. David Miller owner of Group of Forty, wrote "Tachyon energy fulfills a need unmet by crystals for transmutation of life-force energy (Miller).

This book provides teachings and instruction based on the visions I received, and later added research that I found about the energies. They generally describe Tachyon energy in a similar format as to how I received the information.

The energies themselves, when invoked, automatically work within the interdimensional aspects of earth to balance and harmonize the energies in love, light, peace, unity, prosperity, and oneness.

What is Kryon? Some people who have worked with Kryon, refer to it as an angelic being that provides the means for humanity to rise in consciousness and energetic light vibration. Kryon is often channeled here on earth. The first channel was Lee Carroll in the 1980s. Quite a bit can be found about this energy through those who channel Kryon. Most of what I have received through visions and meditations is in alignment with the information I have found through verification of research.

Types of Energies: There are levels for balancing, clearing, investigating, and creating, as we will discuss in the following chapters. The first few chapters are energies that can be used daily. Each group of energies can be quite intense and may take time to master. I recommend a practitioner start by using a few energies, and mastering them before learning others. It is possible that practitioners will find five to six energies that assist them with their healing, and that is all they use. There is no need to master *all* the energies. It is best to work with the energies that call to the healer or are alignment with the work that he or she does.

2 PREPARATION & SELF CARE

Space Preparation

Purpose: When a healer is working in a space it is much easier if the area is clean and pure to bring in the higher levels of light and vibration as well as protection.

Preparing the Space: Any space may be prepared anywhere, and it only takes a few minutes. It is a common practice in the healing arena for highly sensitive empathic healers to prepare all spaces, prior to entering into them. Empaths are so sensitive that they may feel or even be affected by the energies and emotions that existed in the space prior to or while they are there. It is an excellent practice to prepare the energy and set the intentions of the space, prior to entering a meeting, going to a new location, or even entering home or work on a daily basis.

How to prepare a space: Use the mind's eye, or third eye to imagine a vortex below the space to release any "murky", undesired or low vibration emotions or energies from the space. Place an imaginary white dome of light over the space for protection. Imagine any lower vibrational or "murky" looking energies falling into the vortex followed by the space becoming filled with a bright light. Once the space is cleared, imagine that the vortex is closed so as to not drain your energy. Lois Wetzel provided great training on this when I took her training on spiritual healing.

When pulling in energy, always pull it in through the crown chakra and use the universal energy rather than your own. For more information on Chakras see the self – care section.

Once the energies are learned in this book, the twenty four energies may be incorporated into the process for protecting and clearing the space. I would recommend revisiting this page frequently while learning the energies, and after completing the book to learn more advanced ways to clear a space.

Practitioner Self-Care

Daily Preparation: To be able to prepare spaces wherever and whenever needed, a practitioner is wise to keep a high level of self- care. It is recommended to do 20 minutes of self – care each morning to prepare for each day in the morning and before bed including, positive mindset, setting intentions, aura cleansing, energy balancing, tai qi, yoga, and other forms of physical health, mixed with meditation. Gaia has great classes, having a positive teacher and mentor is imperative. Abraham Hicks, Wayne Dyer and other speakers have excellent books and Youtube videos on positive mindset meditations. I highly recommend using these daily when doing any kind of healing work.

Using Yoga in self – care: Yoga aligns your aura with the higher dimensions up to the sixteenth. All forms of yoga are good. Yin or restorative yoga is good for people who have adrenal fatigue or excessive stress. Ashtanga flow is great for those who are more active and energetic and contains a series of poses that align with the higher dimensional energies. Kundalini yoga activates the energy centers and can be a powerful aspect of a practice. Generally people feel calm, balanced, centered and have more clarity after doing yoga. To properly receive the benefits of yoga, it is best to hold each pose for one minute.

Daily Meditations: As mentioned, yoga and other modalities connect to the higher dimensions, as does meditation. The purpose of meditation is to calm the mind and the nervous system and reach the sub conscious mind and the higher divine self. Meditation can be done in standing qigong form or as a sitting form on a chair or in lotus on the floor, the most important thing is to ensure that the feet are touching the floor and the spine is straight, this allows the spine and the energy centers to align with the earth and heavens. Below are best practices for meditations. Most healers are already practicing some form of meditation.

1. **Grounding:** The purpose is to ensure that the meditator is still connected to the earth reality. The risk of not grounding is that they become disconnected by the earthly reality and find it difficult to function in daily life. First, ground yourself by imagining that you have a tree trunk in the center of your body, and the roots are going into the ground, with limbs extending as arms and legs. The yoga tree or mountain poses are excellent for grounding. It is best done in a green space with trees and plants and barefoot. This is the reason that yoga is often performed barefoot and close to the earth.

2. **Protection:** Protecting ones energy while healing is very important. Similar to having a virus protection, it is important that the energy that is being worked with is of the light and highest vibration. When opening up to the higher realms, without proper protection undesirable energies or even entities could enter ones aura. Protect your energy by surrounding yourself and your entire energy body with a white light. When we begin to discuss the energies we will discuss a protection energy called Polykryon. This energy can be activated when doing the protection process of the healer and the client. I will go over this in more detail when we start the energy section.

Types of Meditation:

Dr. Masters from the University of Sedona explains the types of meditation well in the program or metaphysics that I attended. Below is a guideline based on his teachings. Refer to this section regularly as many of the energies will utilize one or the other, or both.

1. **Mystical meditation;** in which the person sits in a quite space, performs breathing exercises and quiets the mind. There are many types of breathing exercises that may be utilized. It is best for the healer to use the method that are most comfortable with. I often recommend to those new to meditation to inhale through the mouth 5 times, hold for the count of 5 and exhale. Really any number of breaths may be utilized. Some practices like to use sacred numbers such as 3, 9 and 12 breaths in their meditations. The more experienced meditator may use more breaths as they feel comfortable. Once the breathing exercises have calmed the mind to a point of stillness, the meditator will receive what comes. Early on the meditator may not be able to stay still for long and may not receive anything. After practicing the length and quality of the meditation will increase. Once they have reached the

point of stillness and complete calm, people will often see images, lights, symbols, or other visions such as angels or ascended masters. Journaling after meditation is an excellent way to record what is seen or felt during the meditation. It is common to forget the experiences after coming out of the meditation and back into the conscious mind.

2. **Manifestation meditation;** a meditation in which the person has a mantra or a desired creation through a thought form. The mantra creates instructions for the subconscious mind. For instance, the healer may say, "I am love, light, peace, unity and oneness, one with God in highest good for healing." These manifestations create the vibration of the body, the aura and the subconscious mind. This is a powerful way to change the conscious and subconscious mind rapidly. This mind programming cannot be done in a conscious state.

Chakra Cleansing and Preparation: Below is a brief overview of the chakra systems, I have listed several excellent books in the reference section, that go into full detail about chakra meditations and clearing for those seeking a deeper understanding.

The chakras have been a part of Eastern Philosophy for thousands of years. The West has begun to adopt the use of them in masses more recently especially with the introduction of yoga and meditation to the west. There are 7 popularly known chakras which we will discuss, and up to 16 that connect with the earth energy centers and higher dimensions. James Tyberonn goes into great detail about earth energy centers and vortices in his books and teachings. Refer to the reference section to learn more.

Chakra Descriptions and use:

- **Seventh, Crown:** This chakra is white in color and is located on the vortex of the head. This chakra connects the person to the infinite God higher self, and moves beyond ego and karma. This chakra is the location where we pull healing energies into our field from the infinite God source, and may release any blockages in connecting to source. When it is out of balance or closed, a person will feel disconnected and separate from God.

- **Sixth, Third Eye:** This chakra is purple in color and is in the location of the third eye or the center of the forehead. This chakra allows us to use our abilities of foresight and intuition also known as the "mind's eye", to see that which cannot be seen with the physical eyes. We will be using this chakra throughout this book for healing and in use with the energies.

 In order to use these energies properly, the third eye will require regular balancing and clarity to ensure that the information received during sessions is clear.
This chakra balances spirituality and brings clarity, connects to guides, and acts as a filter for intuition and guidance. The first three chakras must be in balance and harmony for the third eye to receive clear and balanced information.

- **Fifth, Communication:** This chakra is blue in color and is related to communication. When this chakra is in balance the healer will effectively use sound for healing through music, singing or language in a positive and loving way. A client will have positive communication and a balanced voice. When this chakra is opened, there is power and creativity in the spoken word. The use of this chakra can be powerful in meditations and invocations for several of the energies in this book. In this book we will focus on balancing communication into love, light, harmony, and peace, and releases dysfunction in communication or even lack of communication.

- **Fourth, Heart:** This chakra is located in the center of the chest and is green in color. This chakra is related in mysticism to union with God and the absolute power. The participant will be aligned with the infinite light, and generally the ego self is lost to being in the vibration of oneness when the heart is open. Many yoga poses called heart opening poses help to keep this chakra open and Balanced to the vibration of love, peace, and compassion. Balancing this chakra will release anxiety, stress and feeling overwhelmed.

- **Solar Plexus:** This chakra is yellow in color, is located near the solar plexus where the soul is believed to reside, and also the location of the spleen. When this chakra is open and balanced it will strengthen the healing ability. This chakra balances clarity in soul purpose, divine soul alignment, willpower, and balanced divine feminine and masculine of the soul. Since this is the location of the soul it makes sense that the balance of the divine feminine and masculine will also reside here. We will talk more about this later.

- **Second, Navel:** This chakra is located at the naval area and can be seen as a vibrant orange color. When balanced and open, this chakra connects us with the mind's perception balancing ego and confidence. When first opened, there may be unclear perceptions, however, over time the clarity will improve. Emotionally, this chakra balances confidence, belief in self, ability to take action, humility, creative energy, nurturing and caring for others. Women tend to connect with the nurturing aspect of this chakra and the ability to be fertile especially during the child bearing years.

  When the ego is out of balance, this chakra will also be out of balance. Often the demands on earth from a third dimensional perspective require feeding the earthly desires for power, control and superiority. These are ego based desires. The higher vibrations requires more humility and less ego of power and control. The ego may be balanced in this chakra by releasing issues with power and control, and adding a more balanced healthy confidence, with trust in life and God. Those in fear tend to be out of balance in this chakra and the heart chakra as they will develop anxiety based on their fears. This imbalance will block the ability to work with the energies and provide healing.

- **First, Sacral:** This is the base chakra in the color of red, and is considered the place of awakening or the kundalini energy. When the kundalini is activated it will move up the spine and can open all of the chakras. Working with this chakra, heals issues dealing with safety, security, prosperity, sexual boundaries and trust in the basics of life being provided through God. When this chakra is not functioning properly it will be difficult for a person to function in the other chakras. Many people activate the first and other chakras through kundalini yoga. When basic needs are met and one feels safe and prosperous they are able to connect more easily to source and manifest their desires. When they are out of balance they will be in a state of victim hood and lack which often blocks healing and the ability to use the energies.

Balancing the Chakras

We often think that our aura is limited to our first 7 chakras, however in fact, once we have opened up to the fifth dimension, we have access to align with up to sixteen dimensions or chakras. Once we balance and open up the chakra system, we are open to higher consciousness that allows us to expand our reality. In order to expand this way, first balance the first seven chakras, and open the crown chakra to align to heaven.

Steps for opening and balancing the chakras:

- Prepare the space.
- Imagine each chakra one to sixteen being filled with a great white light.
- Using the mind's eye to imagine that each chakra is turning counterclockwise twelve times.
- Use the mind's eye to determine if there are any blockages in these chakras (dimensions), imagine the white light filling it, and releasing the murky energy into a vortex below the body. I recommend the healer clear the energy body regularly throughout the day or weak depending on the frequency of healing work.
-

- Fill each chakra with the vibrant color associated with the chakra.
- Once this is complete imagine that each is spinning clockwise which is the natural direction of the chakras to spin. This is considered the healthy state.
- One may also close the chakras for protection against unpleasant energies.
- Once the entire energy body is filled with a white light from chakra one to sixteen, surround it again with protection. Please see the references section for a book on the mind's eye, if more information is needed.
- Remember to close the vortex after you have completed the cleansing to conserve your energy.
- Repeat the aura cleansing of the your own energy, after the session as most healers and empaths will pick up the "gunk" of those they are healing.

Other Self-Care

1. It is highly recommended to receive regular healing massages, reflexology, or acupuncture from a practitioner who understands how to balance energy and has a good positive energy that improves the practitioner's energy body.
2. Take regular baths in Epsom salts, lavender oils, and apple cider vinegar, as these will reduce inflammation, pain, emotional and physical toxins out of the physical body and aura.
3. Eat fresh, organic foods with plenty of vegetables, high in minerals and antioxidants.
4. Regular juicing and cleanses or detoxes are recommended to keep the body clear of emotional or physical toxins.
5. Get regular sleep, with naps as needed. Six to eight hours of sleep is recommended per night to keep the circadian rhythms in alignment and allow the physical body, the aura to heal and allow dream-state cellular and mental repair to stay young and healthy.

3 PRACTITIONER ACTIVATIONS

Energy Activations: In order to be activated in using the energies, the practitioner will go through an activation process.

Self- Preparation: Prior to doing an activation prepare the energy body and maintain a high level of self-care.

Sit in a quiet space in a comfortable position for the meditation with the spine straight and ground the feet on the floor or sit on the floor in lotus position with the legs crossed.

- Do a full chakra clearing and balancing prior to the invocation.
- Do a full meditation prior to the invocation and maintain the meditative state during the invocation.
- Prepare a protective energy surrounding the person being activated.

Invocation: This activation need only be done once for each practitioner. It may be completed by a teacher or facilitator of the energies or oneself.

Set the following intention and say the phrases out loud.

I _____ (say your name), hereby acknowledge that I will use the herewith in energies for the highest good of myself, humanity, the planet, and our solar system. My intentions for use of these energies are solely for healing people and the environment in which we live here on this earth. I intend to heal many people and the environment, to create a place of peace, love, unity, oneness and prosperity. I am open to receive the gift of the twenty-four energies and their inherent abilities to heal humanity and earth. I realize that the energies work through me, and I am a conduit of these energies. As a conduit, I agree to remain humble, and provide the credit for the healing, to the energies through the source of the omnipresent God. These energies will work through me, so long as I remain in a vibration of love, light, peace, unity, and oneness. I agree, that I will inform all those I directly work with, that these energies work through me as a higher technology of healing energy. I do not possess special powers as part of this healing, and the gift they receive is the gift of healing from God.

I agree to obtain permission from a person prior to performing a healing on them using these energies. If the person is not open to talking about the energies, I agree to ask the person permission to perform a healing, and use my intuition or guidance to decide if the energies are an acceptable form of healing for this person. I may ask their higher self for permission as an alternative to a verbal request. Thank-you God and the higher angelic realms for bestowing upon me, this gift of healing.

SARA FLORIDA PhD

SACRED GEOMETRY ACTIVATIONS

For the highest benefit of the Sacred Geometry Art, look at them in depth, and meditate with them for deeper activations within you. Sacred Geometry Art is throughout the book to add powerful activations in alignment with the energies.

LOVE

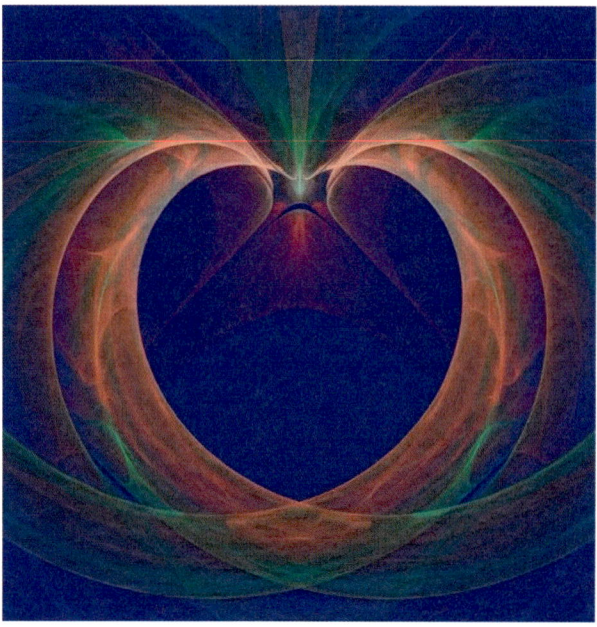

LAW OF GRATITUDE

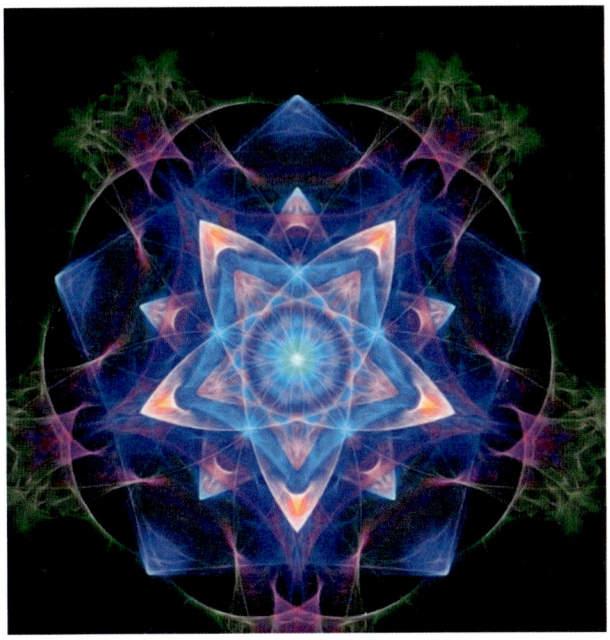

Sacred Geometry by Leon Van Kraayenburg

For the full deck of cards visit: **www.sacreddnakeys.com**

4 INVOKING THE ENERGIES

Space Preparation:

1. Use **Polykryon** energy to create a protection around yourself and the space where the work is being done. This energy will be described in more detail in chapter 4, when we discuss the individual energies.
2. Imagine an energy vortex being placed under the space where the healing will be performed, to absorb any negative or clearing energies that will occur.
3. Enter into a meditative alpha state for invoking the energies.
4. *Generally, the space should be clean, peaceful, and have a high vibration, nice soft music, or relatively quiet, and generally feel good to the healer.* The Law of Attraction states that whatever we pay attention to, we attract.
 If there are distractions, uncomfortable loud noises, or other distractions in the healing space, these could play into the amplification of the energies.

5. If the space has any uncomfortable, "murky", or negative energies, use the clearing energies such as **Claryon** or **Negkryon** (found in the chapter on clearing energies), to clear the space prior to working on a person or performing the other work. It is an excellent practice to clear all spaces before working.
6. Once the work is complete, use the clearing energies once again to clear the space.
7. Use the mind's eye (imagination) to close the vortex under the space once complete.

Invocations for the Human Body

1. **Permission:** Obtain permission from the patient or person being healed to perform the healing process, and ask for "the highest good for the entity to be healed."
2. **Locate the Areas that Need Healing:** The practitioner will scan the space or the body that is being healed for areas of concern using the mind's eye, intuition, and/or using hands, depending on how the practitioner sees energy. Areas of concern will often appear as murky gray or other non vibrant colors in the mind's eye. When using the hands, the area will feel dense and heavy, depleted, or otherwise out of balance.

3. **Determine the problem:** Once the areas of concern have been determined, it is best to use intuition or guidance to understand what type of problem is at hand, so the appropriate energy or energies may be used.
4. **Set the Mode:** Say out loud or in the mind, "I work as a conduit of these healing energies from the God source in a vibration of love, light, peace, unity, and oneness to heal this person."
5. **Set the Intention:** Once the areas and type of energy needed are determined, the practitioner will set the intention of the healing session by stating out loud or in the mind what is the intention of the session, including the intended areas to be healed, and the desired outcome. When practicing, this can be written down.
    Example: "We will clear the energies that are causing anxiety and stress in this person."
6. **Direct the Energy:** The energies work very fast, so after the intention is set, the practitioner will direct the energy to the area that is desired to heal, using the mind's eye.
7. **Invocation:** Repeat three times the name of the energy being activated while sending it to the area being healed with the mind's eye. Say the words, "I invoke this energy across all timelines, all dimensions, past, present, and future."

Invoking Multiple Energies: More than one energy may be used at a time.

For example, if an area requires physical, emotional, and past-life healing, then the three energies will all be activated simultaneously and directed at the area to be healed with the mind's eye. (Individual energies will be detailed in the following chapters with examples.) The healer would invoke: "**Tachyon, Playon, Goryon** across all timelines, all dimension, past, present and future."

Environmental Invocations: If the energy is being invoked to heal something in the environment, such a green space or pollution, there are a few changes to the protocol. Instead of directing the energy toward a person, it will be directed in a dome shape to the area being healed. The invocation is the same.

Permission: Obtain permission from a higher self or ask that the energies be used in the "highest good for all involved."

Time: In the higher dimensions, time does not exist as it does in the third dimension in a linear fashion. When energies are invoked, sometimes results can occur immediately, and other times, they may take time. When I say *time* in linear, third-dimensional time, it could be days, weeks, months, or even years. Most of the time, there will be some indication that a plan is taking shape and changes are beginning to occur. Each energy is different in how it manifests.

For example, when using Tachyon, the energy for physical ailments, it could begin to manifest in that the person receives a strong pain in the digestive system that requires him or her to research the ailment further, by reading or even obtaining some testing for the digestive system. This could lead the person to realize that taking a certain vitamin or mineral will correct the digestive dysfunction.

Sometimes the energies will work and make great changes on their own, and other times the energies will guide the person to a series of events that will cause the healing to occur. I have used this thousands of times for myself and for patients.

For example, I once had a skin condition that I tried many ways to remedy, and it was not healing to my satisfaction. Once I used the energies, I was led through a series of events to determine the healing protocol. The energies help to automatically balance any imbalance that may lead to a condition, and assist with the immediate surroundings to bring what is to be healed into balance. It can manifest in many ways and in multiple timelines and throughout all dimensions, past, present, and future.

In the fifth dimension and higher, all of time exists at one point in the present moment. This is difficult to grasp from a third-dimensional, linear point of view; however, it is the case. When the energies are activated, they can heal the issue in all of time. For example, in the movie, *Back to the Future*, when an action changed, it affected the future. This works the same way. If, when activated, the energy heals a situation from the past, it will affect the current situation as well as the future.

Examples: When invoking the energy for creating green space, **Pimikryon**, whether this person is planning to do gardening or not, the energy will invoke the energy to create a green space. Sally may invoke this energy in a place that has no green, and she may find that the city initiates plans to create a new green space in the location where she invoked the energy. A second example:

perhaps a neighbor fails to take care of his yard, leaving the street looking less than desirable. If the energy is invoked on that yard, it will be amazing to see that within higher-dimensional time and reality, that yard will be transformed. Perhaps you will see the neighbor suddenly takes initiative to care for his yard, or he hires a landscaper. The energy works in ways that are not easily understood by the third-dimensional linear mind. I have witnessed this many times. Living in Houston, I frequently drive down polluted and unkempt streets. (Many streets are beautiful and full of trees.) When I travel on these streets, I will often invoke the energies, and I am always pleased by the eventual transformation of these areas. I have done the same on my own street, which is an older street with houses built in the 1960s. Since I have invoked the energies on my street, six houses on the street have been remodeled and made to have much higher vibration and beauty.

Intent: When working with the energies, it is best to set a positive intention of the outcome that you would like to occur.

Manifestation and Allowing: It is best to invoke the energies with an intention of allowing. Our mind-set will influence the outcome, a positive mind-set with full trust that our manifestation will occur, will bring about the highest and good. We invoke the energy, create our manifestation, allow and trust. We allow with confidence, with patience, and from a place of peace. If we are working on patients, it is wise to train them to "allow" the healing to occur as it does. Give them the expectation that all will occur in the divine timing, on a nonlinear scale. Anxiety, stress, and impatience will block the energies and the manifestations. Again, remember: *manifest our creations in peace, and allow in patience.*

Patient State of Consciousness: Generally, it is necessary to use these energies on healing subjects who are vibrating in the fifth dimensional level or above realm. This will require a level of intuition and knowing from the healing practitioner. If you are unsure about this, I highly recommend studying the characteristics of the fifth dimensional consciousness further before proceeding with the energies. Many books are listed in the references section at the end of this book.

When the consciousness is in the higher dimensions, the energies are more likely to work on the patient. I have been guided to focus these energies on these higher-vibrating patients for the sheer reason that their energy bodies will be compatible with the energies. This requirement is only the case with humans. If they are not ready for this level of healing, it could be a shock to the system. It would be like bringing in HD television to a tube television. Objects and spaces are capable of receiving the energies.

5 PHYSICAL AND EMOTIONAL HEALING ENERGIES

These energies are the basis for the twenty-four energies and are used most frequently. They are used to heal emotions and physical space that are directly observable in our current situation, spaces around us or patients. They can all be used by themselves, or in combination with any other energy in this book. I highly recommend learning the energies in this chapter first, and becoming comfortable with them prior to learning the other energies.

Guided versus Automatic Healing

Automatic: Each of the energies are capable of healing, using the invocation process with little or no guidance from the practitioner other than setting the intention of the energy and allowing. The healer may choose the energies needed for the healing and invoke multiple energies at one time.

Guided: Use the mind's eye to see or feel energies, and guide the energy appropriately. The healer will be more actively involved in the healing session, and have more insight as to what further energies need to be invoked for the healing. If the person being healed is open to it, the healer may share what is occurring.

1. **POLYKRYON**

Protection: This energy is the most important in the twenty-four energies and is to be invoked every time any of the energies are used. It is used as protection while doing work and throughout the day. It appears as a shimmering platinum yet clear color. This energy is the one to be used during preparation and anytime practitioners feel they need to protect their energy. The purpose of the protection is to provide a shield from any forces that may reside in the surrounding space, timelines, or dimensions that are not in the highest good of the work. It is important to invoke this energy in a feeling of love, light, safety, and security. If there are any fearful feelings, it is best to avoid using the energies.

Use: During invocation, imagine that the platinum shimmering energy is surrounding the practitioner's energy body as well as the energy body of the person or the area to be healed. This can be done multiple times in a session or throughout the day as needed. Review the invocation process for the full invocation of this energy in conjunction with the other energies.

BALANCE

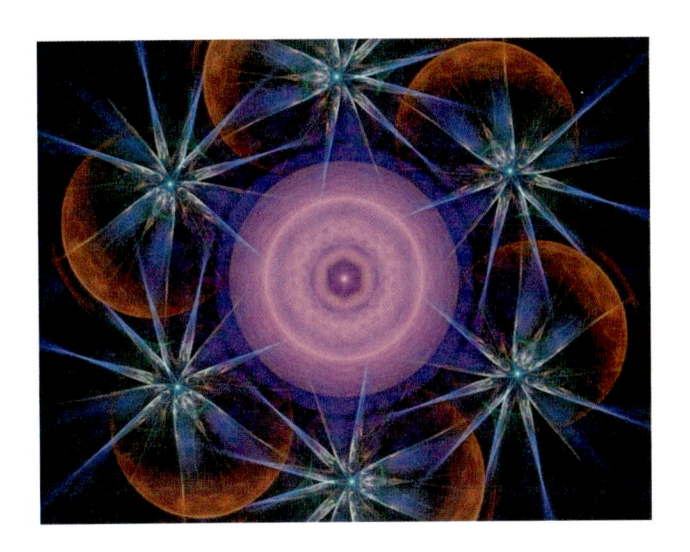

2. TACHYON

Physical ailments; this energy balances physical manifestations and is already well known on earth. It is an energy that is like a white shimmering platinum color that vibrates faster than the speed of light. The purpose of this energy is to clear physical health ailments and pain. It does so by creating a vibration faster than the physical pain or ailment and transmuting it back into health.

Use: Follow the invocation we have learned previously and focus attention on the area of the body that is inflicted with poor physical health or pain. Imagine this platinum shimmering energy engulfing this space. This energy, like the others, will balance and begin the healing process automatically; there is no need to do additional balancing work for this area of the physical body. It can be used in conjunction with other healing modalities such as acupuncture, massage, herbs, oils, etc. It is not recommended to combine this with other forms of energy works outside of the twenty four energies, (such as reiki), as it stands alone. It is best to do the other forms of healing first and then apply the Tachyon energy to complete the process.

Healing from Tachyon energy, like the others, is automatic and may come in many forms. It may lead a person to seek out a new kind of healing they had not thought of before, it may assist the individual with guidance for the perfect remedy, or it may heal the person at that time. These occurrences could be through divine intervention, such as a friend suddenly talking about it or a stranger telling the person about a herbal remedy. As we discussed, allow time to manifest in the divine fifth-dimensional nonlinear time. The person will usually feel relief and may report experiencing interesting and unexpected healing. Tachyon will provide or guide a person to the highest healing for his or her condition.

Healing Etiquette: Do not interfere with this process by giving excessive advice to the person beyond providing the healing during the initial session. It is beneficial to the process to check in with the person about his or her healing regularly and ask about progress. Allow for the energies to work and guide you and the patient to what steps will be next. You may hear some interesting and profound stories. Tachyon may be used multiple times until the healing is complete, but be sure to allow it to do its work. Overuse and anxiety about the outcome could block the energies.

If individuals are not open to the use of the energy, they are not of the vibration to use it, so it is best not to use it on them. There are many other subtler healing modalities available for this case. I have used this energy most commonly with the most outstanding results. This energy has been received and used by others on this planet, so this book is not the first introduction. I have reviewed their work, after using it for quite some time, and it has given validation to me, about the use of the energies.

3. PLAYON

Playon is the energy that balances the emotional body. This energy looks like a thin, ray of thin and nearly transparent crystalline light in multiple colors according to the chakra colors.

Use: The best use of it is to identify the emotions that need to be released and focus this energy to the part of the body or the part of the earth where these emotions are residing. Use the mind's eye to see the energy of the area to be healed and determine the color of the emotion to be released. The color chart is listed below.

Invocation: Repeat the word *Playon* three times and allow. This energy is automatic and will create release and balancing on its own, so there is no need to focus on the healing for an extended time. Invoke the energy, and allow it to do its work.

This energy is automatic. However, if a specific area of the body or the aura is being worked on or a certain emotion, the following colors may be guided to the area for clearing or reinforcing by imagining the area being filled with the appropriate color. Release the non-vibrant or murky colors and direct the new vibrantly colored energy to the area.

Aura/Chakra Colors: Negative and Positive :

- White: Clears sadness, depression, disconnectedness from spirit and source

- Purple: Clears clutter and blockages to spirituality and intuition

- Blue: Clears blockages in communication or negativity in communication

- Green: Clears anger, disgust, judgment, anxiety, and indecision of the heart, issues of not feeling connected, and lack of love

- Yellow: Clears worry, confusion, and self-doubt, lack of direction, issues related to self-will and disharmony between masculine and feminine

- Orange: Clears negative excessive ego triggers, inaction, laziness, issues with confidence, creative blockages, and infertility

- Red: Clears lack and fear, insecurity, issues related to being grounded, and safety-related issues

Use the chakra system to rebalance the emotions. Begin with the first chakra, to rotate the chakra counterclockwise and release all that no longer serves, and do this for each. Activate the energy on each chakra while they are open. Imagine the energy flowing out of each until you see that all the negative vibration energies have been released. The energy will automatically release the negative and replace the positive.

For those not familiar with the chakra system, this is only a brief overview, I recommend studying this further prior to using the energies. I have provided a brief overview of the chakra system in the self- care chapter of this book as well as a few excellent books on advanced chakra healing in the reference section of this book.

6 CLEARING ENERGIES

The purpose of these energies is to clear out that which no longer serves us in the form of emotions, blockages, energies and more. These can be used in people, objects, or spaces. Healer's typically require regular clearing of their energy, workspaces and clients. It is important for us to stay clear so that the work we do has more clarity and the energy moving into the space or the client is pure.

4. CLARYON

Clarity and release of clutter: This energy is best used when we have a cluttered mind or space. It is beneficial when we notice that we are receiving multiple mixed messages, manifestation is not as fast or clear as usual, our intuition is unclear, we have a hard time making decisions, we feel overwhelmed, or feel ill at ease with our surroundings because of too much clutter.

Use: To invoke this energy, follow the invocation steps; identify which areas of life, mind, or space need clearing or clarity, and call out the name three times, saying *Claryon*; then allow it to manifest. This is an automatic energy requiring no further action.

Manifestation: Results can range from immediate to several weeks. You will feel a shift and receive spiritual and intuitive guidance on what needs clearing. You may ask, *If I have no clarity, how will I receive the guidance?* The answer is that the energy will assist in making this information clear for you. This can range from guidance from your guides to releasing objects from your home or work space, releasing tasks or thoughts that are cluttering your mind, or even a recommendation to balance your energy body.

It is best to do a daily five-minute meditation with journaling to receive the messages necessary to carry out the actions. The energy may balance some of your thoughts and energies for you automatically. It may be necessary for you to do some balancing yourself during your meditations and using the chakras, so you may be aware of the healing process and change related thoughts, feelings, habits or behaviors that are no longer serving you.

5. NEGKRYON

Release negativity: This energy is used to release negativity from the human and earth energy bodies. Imagine it as a vacuum that is sucking out negative gray or murky energies. It can be used on a person's energy body or any space on earth. When it is determined that negative energies are present, follow the space preparation and invocation process. Invoke Negkryon energy and direct it toward the negativity that you wish to be released. The negativity can be a thought, a belief, a situation, or a space.

Use: Imagine the negative energies being sucked up through a vacuum hose into the vortex that was created. This energy is automatic like the others and need only be invoked with intention and then allow it to do its work. Once the session is complete and the mind's eye sees that the negative energies are clear, close the vortex.

This energy is often used in conjunction with **Playon Energy** to balance the emotions. Negkryon will release the negativity, and Playon will balance them.

Patient Care: The energy will continue to work after the session is complete, so it is good to advise the patient to take a nice bath in Epson salts or apple cider vinegar to assist with the release, and be aware that his or her emotions may feel strong for a few days while they are clearing. The patient can be advised to get extra rest and inform family members and friends that he or she is doing emotional work and that strong emotions may suddenly arise. The patient could journal and keep in touch via e-mail or phone, to let the practitioner know how the patient is feeling.

6. ANKRYON—(Ankh)

Clear imbalances in feminine and masculine: This ancient symbol of life and fertility represents the balance of the male and female. The Egyptian cross is a powerful energetic tool for eternal life. The ankh symbol can be used energetically to balance the divine feminine and divine masculine through clearing imbalances and unification. This harmonization into perfect union is essential to raising the vibration and eternal life of the soul.

Use: This energy is most appropriate when an energy body needs balancing of the divine feminine and masculine to equality. The use of this energy will increase the vibration of the energy body and open the energy body up to rapid growth and expansion.

To use the Ankryon energy, imagine the ankh over the chakra being worked on, and follow the invocation process. Use the mind's eye to place this symbol on the energy body, and it will perform the work of the energy. It may be placed on one chakra or all sixteen.

7. PIMIKRYON

Clearing, balancing, and healing green spaces: This energy can be used in a space of any size. It is best to use it in a space that is easy to see in the mind's eye or imagination.

Examples: These may include a garden in the backyard, healing a forest, or maybe even an area that lacks green space and needs it in the middle of a city.

Use: Set the intention of what is to occur in the area, imagine the space as it is, and place an imaginary white platinum energy dome over the space. Imagine it converting into the beautiful green space that it could be by using the invocation process to invoke the energy.

How it works: This energy does not require the practitioner to perform anything physical. The practitioner does not need to hire a team of landscapers and develop a budget to make this work. The energy will occur on its own.

Example: say I were to invoke the energy in a downtown area over a space that is desired to heal, clear or balance. I later return to the space, perhaps weeks or months later. A local developer has decided to remodel a building and add a small park to the area. If I did this at my home and lacked the time to do it myself, within a period of time, perhaps my neighbor would come over and offer to weed my yard and plant new plants free of charge if I provide plants. (That is a true story.)

Time: Like the other timeframes we talked about, the time will be according to the universal plan. When you do the invocation, ask that it be done according to the divine plan, and it will. This could be days, weeks, months, or years in linear, 3-D time. The important part is to invoke and allow. Check back to see the progress.

7 INVESTIGATIVE ENERGIES

These energies are best used for investigation, researching, or finding out answers related to the necessary healing. This is a more advanced form of healing for the seasoned healer. These energies are useful in healing a person, place or thing, when we must first determine why it is out of balance in the first place. These energies can be used for cases that are less obvious and require deeper understanding for the healing to occur.

For example, if someone came to a healer for healing of a pain and had an obvious injury, this would have a cause and no need for deeper answers. However, if a person came to the healer and had a lifetime of pain in an area of the body that had no explanation, no doctor could find any reason for the pain, this would be a reason to do further investigation to determine the underlying cause. Typically, this energy is useful if the energies for balancing and clearing have not completely healed the issues at hand. Healers who use these energies typically have a form of connection with the divine, in which they are able to receive information from the subconscious of the earth plane, humanity, multidimensionality, or across all timelines.

Methods to Receive Answers Using These Energies

Automatic: The energy is invoked, and it clears on its own without the information entering into the conscious mind of the healer or the patient. Neither will be aware of what occurred or healed. However, in the multidimensional divine timeline, changes and healing will occur.

Guided: The practitioner may access this information for the person or guide him or her to receive the information by going into a meditative state. This option will be based on the capabilities of the healer and the willingness or openness of the patient. Both the healer and the patient will become aware of the incidents that occurred and will be healed. The healer will say aloud or write through automatic writing, the information that is received during the session. It is a common practice to use a voice recording for the session and provide it to the patient.

Guided Method 1: Automatic Writing will require going into a meditative or alpha state to receive the information. The healer and the person being worked on can use breathing exercises to reach this state. If the person being worked on is comfortable doing so, he or she can perform the automatic writing. If the person is not comfortable doing the automatic writing, the healer may do the automatic writing for him or her. I only recommend this for healers who have experience doing this type of work. This takes practice and study on the part of the healer.

How automatic writing works: Have a pen in hand with blank paper while going into the meditative state. It is best to use a book or multiple sheets of paper, so as to not break the flow state during the process. The healer will receive the information and allow it to flow through the pen without thinking about what is being said. They will write whatever comes into their mind. The writing could occur over one session or multiple sessions if needed. Oftentimes the handwriting will not be the same as the person's normal handwriting, and it could even be difficult to decipher. Once it is clear that the session is complete and no more information is coming, the healer and patient can read the information to determine how it can assist in the healing process.

Guided Method 2: Imagery through Meditation, occurs when the healer goes into a meditative alpha state and guides the patient. There are many ways to do this, so I recommend the practitioner use the method he or she is most comfortable with. The healer can receive images for the person and say them out loud or write them or, if capable, the patient may allow images to flow into her mind's eye while in the meditative state, so that she will see the answers that are requested.

Sharing: It is not necessary for the practitioner to share everything that comes up in the session, if it would make the patient feel uncomfortable. There may be instances when the information that comes up is so traumatic or painful that it is best to simply clear it rather than invoke the energy into the conscious mind of the person being healed. If the person being healed is not completely open to the information that will come up, it is best to use the automatic form and allow it to heal on its own. As long as the person has given permission for healing, the healing can be performed.

Timing: The answers may come at different times however, unlike the other energies, these energies tend to be more instantaneous. Often the answers will come immediately while in a meditative state. If they do not, the person will continue to go into regular meditative states until the answers come to them. The reason this is instantaneous is because the answers already exist in the multidimensional level and only need to be received. timing is based more on the receptive ability of the healer or person seeking the answers.

8. LORYON

Lost Language or Words: This energy is most beneficial when someone is lacking the words for what he or she is trying to say. Often people will say something like, "I have lost the words" or "there are no words to describe it." These thoughts are frequently at a multidimensional level, and the person is unable to access the words or the language because the thought is residing at a different level of consciousness than the spoken third-dimensional language.

Use: Invoke this energy using the regular process, then ask the person to set the intention of the words that he or she wishes to retrieve. Use one of the reception methods above to retrieve the lost words. This energy is directly related to the fifth chakra of communication and sound. Sound healing using Tibetan or crystal bowls, drumming, singing, chanting, invocations or other sound healing are encouraged to be used with this energy. This energy is self-balancing and will work on it's own.

9. FORKRYON

Making Decisions: As the name indicates, this energy is most useful when there is a decision or a "fork in the road." The patient is seeking answers to decisions.

Use: There are multiple steps to using this energy. First, write down the possible outcomes of the decisions, and use the third-dimensional decision making strategies such as a comparison of pros and cons, prior to invoking the energy. Once the analysis is complete, both the healer and the subject will go into the meditative state, and use the invocation process to set the intention of the information that is desired.

For retrieval of answers, use either the "**visionary meditation**" method to view the possible outcomes of the decision or the "automatic writing" method, to write down the potential outcomes. Finally, when receiving the outcomes, place one hand on the heart and feel how the decision feels in the heart. The decision is best made, based on the compilation of the received information, the analysis and the feeling in the heart. The right decision will "feel right", and be clear. Repeat the process until the decision is clear.

Negative emotions related to decisions: When a decision brings up any feelings of negativity, funny feelings, hesitation, anxiety, or upset in the gut, pay attention and ask for clarification to these feelings. The feelings may need clearing, and it would be best to explore them further by using the energies for balancing and clearing, prior to making the decision. When a decision brings up these feelings, it does not necessarily mean it is completely wrong. It may mean the person has a blockage or area that needs healing prior to making the decision.

Example: A person is debating if she should visit her long-lost parents, that would require her travel by airplane. The parents have written a long letter talking about how much they would love to see her. We know that there will be a positive reception on the other hand. While going through the decision process, it is determined that she has an anxiety about traveling on a plane, which stems from the loss of a family member on an airplane at an early age. The feeling has nothing to do with seeing the parents. Once the true cause of the feeling is determined, this fear can be eliminated, so the real decision can be made. Now we ask the question again, "Should she go visit her long-lost parents?" In the process, anxiety may also come up about seeing them for the first time. All the negative emotions would be addressed prior to making the decision. Once the fear of airplanes is addressed and anxieties about seeing the parents are cleared, the person is able to make a decision based on what her heart wants. After looking deeply, receiving some answers and feeling her heart, she decides that she would love to meet them. She may find that her heart yearns to meet her parents, and she is willing to overcome the obstacles in order to do that.

A good decision will feel good, positive, energetic and enthusiastic, with a mood of being ready for action. Repeat the clearing process until the answer feels this way.

10. SLEPLYON

Dream State: During the dream state, we create, we learn, we travel to many places, we heal, and we regenerate. Invoke this energy before falling asleep, for best results, when important answers, healing, or mental cleansing is needed. We often process our subconscious mind in our dreams.

Use: This may be taught to a client to use, or used by the healer for themselves. Set the intentions of what the participant would like to learn by journaling or meditating. Use the invocation process before falling asleep, and go into a meditative state when falling asleep. It is important to invoke the protection before all the energies are used; however, it is especially important before using the dream-state energy. During sleep, we are unable to protect ourselves consciously. This will ensure that no unwanted energies interrupt the process.

Positive Mindset: When using this energy, it is recommended that the healer and the participant do positive mindset meditations for setting positive intentions for the outcomes of the dreams. Refrain from using this energy when the mind is less than positive as negativity such as anxiety, fear or stress will have a negative result on the dream state. It is wise to place a bowl of Himalayan salts in a bowl under the bed to absorb any negativity during this process and be sure to create the vortex for clearing.

Recording: When awakening, have a journal nearby to write down any and all that you remember from the session and journal any changes that occur during the following weeks because of the session. It is recommended that the sessions be invoked on average once per week, with a maximum of three times, if there is a time when quite a bit of trauma or negativity is coming up that needs clearing.

11. GORYON

Past Lives: This energy is best used when it is determined that a person is afflicted by incidents from a past life that are affecting his or her present life, emotionally, physically, spiritually, or intellectually.

Use: Choose either guided or automatic retrieval.

Invocation: Use the standard invocation process and retrieval methods. If using the automatic method, this is all that is required. For a guided retrieval, follow the process and once the past life is revealed or the incidents leading up to the blockage are seen, release the past life trauma and incidents that no longer serve the client. The healer will require the ability to intuit or feel past lives in order to utilize this energy.

Releasing: Imagine the traumas or incidents of the past life as a gray, dirty energy sinking into a vortex below the client. Imagine the person or consciousness being whole and healed in the area that was affected by the past life. Fill the client with a vibrant white light that fills any areas that were released. When setting the intention, acknowledge both the trauma that is to be healed as well as the intended outcome. Once complete, close the vortex and allow the energy to manifest the outcome.

Example: a person is having a financial difficulty, he consistently receives his paycheck and spends it all quickly, leaving him with no money and large amounts of debt from using credit cards. After carefully looking at his life patterns, he has determined that nothing has occurred in his present life, such as childhood beliefs, that could lead to this behavior, so he seeks to find out what is causing it. While doing the session, the practitioner through "visionary meditation", determines that there may be a past-life incident involved. The healer activates the energy to clear the past issue and the client can now move forward with the healing. After the healing and in divine timing, the patient may become more sensible with money and set aside a certain percentage of it, without frustration or anxiety. He may also find that a series of events occurs that forces him to become better with his money.

Automatic versus guided session: It is not necessary to retrieve the past life trauma, if it is determined the trauma is based on a past life, simply invoke the energy and allow it to heal the past life. If preferred, you may use the guided method, which allows more insight to the patient from an analytical point conscious of view, but it is not necessary to perform the healing.

12. GNOSKRYON

Access the book of knowledge: Investigate for karma, phobias, fears, and anxieties in all timelines and all dimensions. Use this energy in combination with **Goryon,** as there is often a tie to past lives. This is helpful when a person is having a blockage to expanding or shifting. It can be valuable when the client feels stuck or is having anxiety about a situation in life. The client may have a belief that was ingrained into the subconscious, which is blocking him.

Use: The practitioner and client will go into a meditative state and use one of the methods for retrieval. The invocation of the energy may clear the blockages using the automatic or the guided methods of retrieval.

Retrieval Method: The automatic method is much faster, and may be the preferred method for use with this energy. Using the guided method may bring the thought to the conscious mind and manifest subconscious issues into the current life, whereas the automatic method will release the trauma without affecting the conscious mind or life.

Invocation: Set the invocation with the focus on the fear, anxiety, or situation that is to be cleared, and ask "that the highest good occur to clear this situation."

8 VIBRATION RAISING ENERGIES

Energies in this chapter are used to raise the vibration of a person, place, community or humanity. As a collective, humanity has made many shifts in vibration over the past few hundred years. Over the past 100 years and especially since the year 2000, the speed at which our vibration is increasing is phenomenal. Similar to the way our technology is always updated and becomes obsolete, the human vibration is constantly shifting upward.

DIVINITY

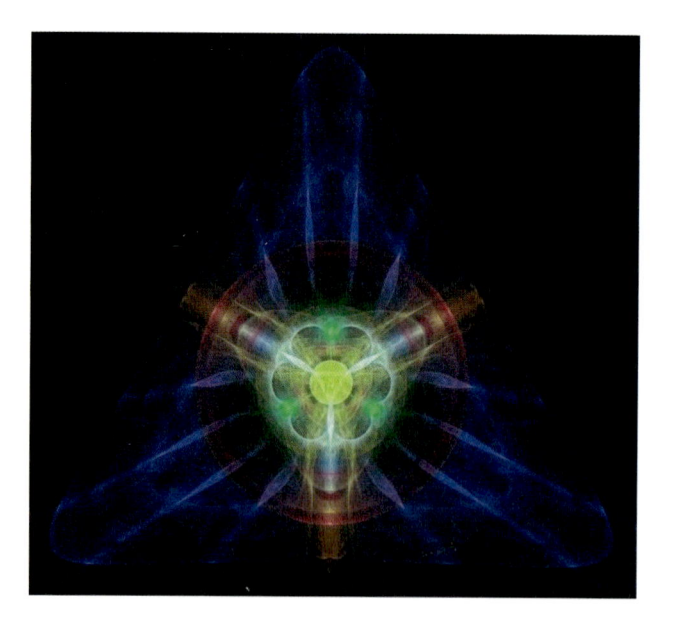

13. COLKRYON

Collective Conscious: This is the energy of healing the collective conscious. There are many reasons to use this. Over time, humanity has created many things. Some creations have served us well, and may have seemed like good ideas at the time, however the long term effects of these ideas have created problems on earth that are not in our highest good. These energies will clear any thought forms, circumstances, situations or things we have created here on earth that no longer serve us in the divine highest good.

Use: To use this energy, set the intent of connecting human consciousness with that of the vibrations of love, light, peace, unity, oneness and highest good. In order to do this, the practitioner must be aligned and in tune with these higher vibrations.

To set the intention, first determine the conscious thoughts, behaviors and actions that are prevalent in society that no longer serve the collective conscious and invoke the **Colkryon** energy. Once the conscious thoughts that are desired to be released are determined, then imagine the consciousness, thoughts, behaviors or actions that will take its place, and ask the **Colkryon** to transform the conscious in the higher good of humanity.

Use it to release fear, hate, rage, corruption violence and so much more. Always imagine the desired outcome with a replacement energy such as peace, love, safety etc. Imagine how it will feel. Emoting the manifestation is an important part of allowing it to come into reality. Abraham Hicks has many Youtube videos and books about the importance of feeling something in order for it to manifest into reality. If we strongly hate something we can manifest more of what we hate. Instead it is better to focus on what we love and want more of. Where we place our focus and our attention is where we manifest and create. For this reason, according to Abraham's teachings, we must carefully monitor what we pay attention to. When we are doing this work, it is good to utilize the daily mindset meditations, set our positive intentions and mind what media we are exposing ourselves to.

Example Invocation "Release the collective conscious energy of fear that is prevalent in our society today into one of peace and higher vibration of love." Imagine, if masses of humanity used this energy daily to heal our planet, the rapid changes that would occur.

Imagine a divine light dome encompassing humanity and releasing fear into a vortex, and use emotions of the heart chakra to feel humanity being at peace.

14. PISTEUYON

Earth Heartbeat: The earth heartbeat is tuned to the universal heartbeat of God. When humanity is aligned with higher vibrations and in harmony with the earth heartbeat, humanity is at peace. The activation of this energy will align the person, group, or community with the earth and God heartbeat of peace, unity, love, oneness, and prosperity.

Use: This energy can be used to heal situations when the patient is feeling overly stressed, anxious. overwhelmed and generally out of alignment with the earth balance. This energy is highly effective when doing work with the fourth heart chakra as it relates directly to the heart and love vibration of God, which aligns with the heartbeat of the earth.

One of the current modern issues related to the changing and increasing level of vibration of humanity is the increase in stress and anxiety that humanity is suffering from. Many people are not able to handle the stress related to the changes and the shifts and they are not aware or trained in methods to manage their energy or stress levels. This energy is one that will help to calm these people down by aligning their heart beat with that of the earth.

15. SANGYON

Sound Healing: Known as the song of light. This energy is used to provide sound healing and raise the vibration using sounds to increase light. This energy will balance, heal, and amplify the sound frequencies of a person, space, area, or even the planet. Sound healing may help ailments, emotions, or situations that bring discordance to the physical, emotional or spiritual bodies.

Use: Many healers use sound healing to work with the vibration of spaces and the energy of the body for healing. Gongs, crystal bowls, drumming circles, and music of all types are popular for healing and balancing the energy body. When used properly, sound and music are extremely healing. When a person is in the presence of discordant sounds, they can disrupt the energy flow in the body, a space, or the earth frequencies.

When using this energy, it is ideal to have a high-frequency sound from either a gong or a Tibetan or crystal bowl to assist with the healing. It is important to invoke the energy when the sounds in the presence of the invocation are of a high frequency with little or no other sound around. This energy primarily works with the fifth chakra of communication and is ideal for balancing this chakra.

Example: Invoking this energy on a noisy freeway or at an airport near planes taking off, would project that sound energy and increase it, so it is best to use this one during a meditative state in the presence of a beautiful high-frequency sound. It can be used to balance noisy areas or sounds, even from a distance. For instance, if there were an unpleasantly noisy area near a patient's home, perform the invocation in a private and pleasant-sounding area, and set the intention to project the pleasant sound into the area with the unpleasant sound.

Space Preparation: Many of the other energies could be invoked in many spaces, however, this energy is important to invoke in a quiet place where the sound is controlled. The preparation is highly important, as whatever occurs in the space related to sound, can be amplified into the healing.

Intention and Clearing: The order of intention is important for this energy. If there are discordant energies or sounds to be cleared, first clear the space using the clearing energies discussed in the earlier chapters. Direct these clearing energies at the area to be healed. After clearing the sounds, set the intention of the energy or sound that the healer would like to amplify. Sound and instruments are the best method for setting the intention using—gong, bowl, music, singing, humming, or whistling. If silence is desired, use complete silence.

16. SALVYON

Infinity Energy: This energy implies salvation into the infinite eternity, which is essentially the goal of many people on earth. This involves raising ourselves and our planet to a higher vibration that is sustainable for eternity. Our light bodies and our planet will continue to rise to higher dimensions and frequencies. Humanity is awakening now in masses of millions per month. There are thousands who have anchored the light one earth, these 144,000 light-workers have heralded in this time of increased vibration for humanity. We are now at a time of critical mass, and the for front of the masses awaking, for the first time in thousands of years, and humanity is moving into the higher vibrations of love, light, peace, unity, prosperity, and oneness.

Humanity have evolved on earth in outstanding leaps in only a few hundred years. This is a time of quickening and an opportunity to ascend into the fifth dimension and beyond. The purpose of this energy is to assist all of humanity in this process.

When invoked, this energy will raise the vibration and consciousness of humanity incrementally. This incremental increase in vibration and consciousness of humanity has been occurring for quite some time on earth. Let me note that the work is being done by the light-workers even without this energy, however this energy will help to amplify the work. The increases in vibration for humanity have been accelerating. Activations have been occurring over the past century, and in increasing numbers of upward shifts each year since 2012 when all of humanity had the ability to awaken. Each human is on their own path and has free will to choose to awaken or not at their own pace. The process could take twenty or more years. It is now quickening at a pace so rapid that the daily changes are astounding.

INFINITE

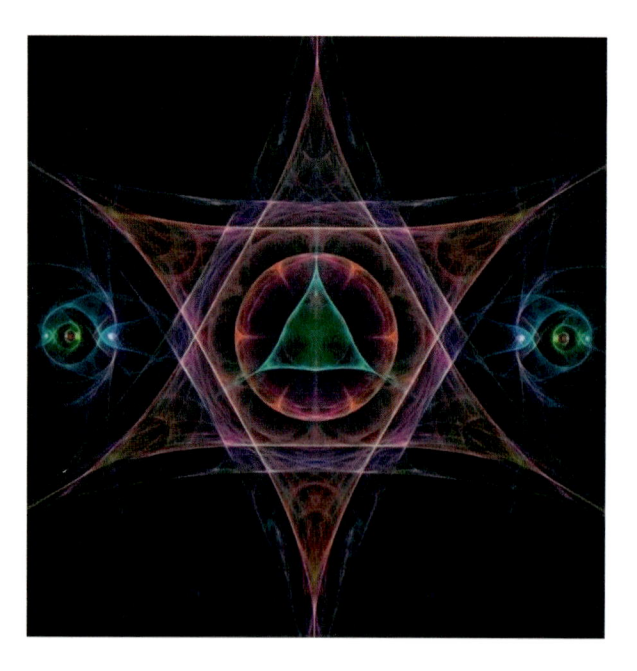

Use: To use this energy, set the intention of raising the vibration of a certain number of people, such as a neighborhood, a community, a city, or even a country. Imagine that area or group of people being enveloped in a white, shiny dome of light, and then imagine that they have increased by the level of vibration indicated. Use a percentage such as ten, or twenty percent.

Invocations that are too intense may not work or could cause an overload of energy upon those located in the area. Energy-overload symptoms include dizziness, fatigue, nausea, and a general feeling of being out of balance. This will only last a short while, one to four days; however, it is best to maintain a lower vibration increase to avoid this. All humans have free will, so it may not affect everyone however, the general rise in vibration of the area will be noticeable where the energy is being used. Use the invocation process and allow. Follow up on your work by releasing attachment to the outcome, and watch for news articles, community changes, and even city changes that indicate the area has shifted to a higher vibration.

9 CREATION ENERGIES

These energies are more advanced, as we discussed earlier. Generally, these energies are used by healers who are guided to do this type of work for humanity or the earth. The vibration for this work will only operate in the vibration of love, light, peace, unity, prosperity, and oneness in alignment with the divine God plan.

Generally, these energies work on a mass or global level, although the intention could be set only to work on a certain area of the planet. Similar to the other energies, the practitioner will set an intention for what is to be created, upgraded or transitioned. Focus the energy on the intention of what is to be created rather than what it is clearing or replacing. There is a method to clear that which is no longer serving us. We will discuss this shortly.

Abraham Hicks and Wayne Dyer have many talks about co-creating and manifesting. I highly recommend listening to these and other positive mindset speakers daily, when working with these energies, in order to keep the mind positive and clear.

CREATION

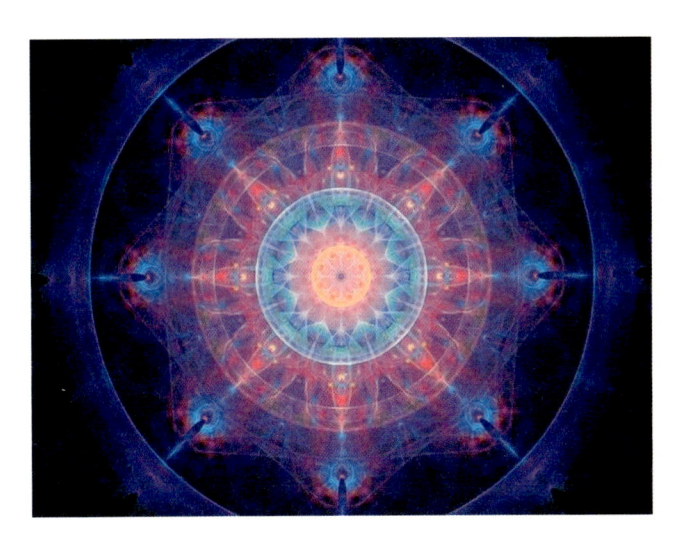

Invoking this energy while being in a pure meditative and positive state, brings about the highest results. When invoking the energy state, *"For the highest good for humanity and the mother earth and in alignment with God"* at the end of every intention. We as humans are quite smart; however, even with best intentions, we are not always aware of the highest good and divine God plan. This will allow for the energy to access the higher interdimensional levels and the angelic realms to create the highest good in a way that we cannot even perceive or fathom from our perspective here on earth.

17. ALPHAKRYON

Beginning: Use this energy for new beginnings. There are many reasons why we may want to set an intention for new beginnings. This will wipe the slate clean and make a fresh start. This can be used for mind-sets, emotional states, processes, and so many other aspects of the human existence.

BEGINNING CREATION

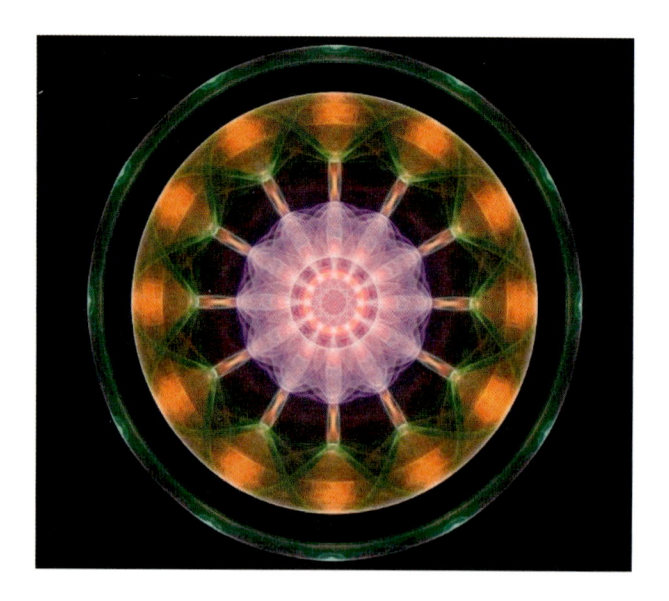

Use: For those guided to do this work, first meditate on what is being restarted and carefully prepare the intention prior to invoking this energy. Once invoked, always remember to add "for the highest good for humanity and the Mother Earth" to the intention. Focus on positive outcomes that vibrate in the higher dimensions.

Use this energy in pair with **Omegakryon** (ending energy) for the best results. In many cases, something must end prior to a new beginning. For instance to end poverty and begin prosperity, one would say: "**Omegakryon** poverty on earth, **Alphakryon** prosperity on earth." This is a big task in our current conditions on earth, so it may take time in the linear world for this invocation to work. It is good to do large global invocations, but also small measurable invocations will allow the healer to see more instantaneous results. In any case the results can be profound. Please note that the invocations will work when they are invoked in the highest good for humanity, earth and in alignment with the divine plan of God. Release attachments to the outcome and allow in the nonlinear fifth dimensional time free from expectations.

Example: I have used these energies for small personal healing sessions as well as global. One day I used the energies to invoke equality for women by saying: **Alphakryon** equality for women in all ways to men on this earth plane". I also used **Omegakryon** in this invocation by saying: **Omegakryon** all ways in which women are unequal to men." A short time after the invocation, there were many items showing up in the news about women demanding rights and where global women rights were changing. These are the energies working through God for the transition of humanity into the higher vibrations. Part of that transition is all humans becoming as one and seen as equal parts.

18. HELIKRYON

Sun Energy: The sun is a vital energy source for humanity. It provides light, energy, and life for earth and humanity. This energy can be used to increase the light in an area. If there are areas of darkness on earth needing energy, warmth, light, and life, this energy can be used to heal these spaces.

Use: Invoke the energy to the area needing healing and allow.

Example: An area of the sea life and corral are dying, this energy could be invoked to this area to begin healing, and restore the natural balance of the ocean. The invocation: "**Helikryon, Helikryon, Helikryon** the healing of the oceans near Australia to restore life to the coral reef in the highest good for all life in that area and in alignment with the highest divine good."

19. MENEKRYON

Moon: The moon brings us light at night and balances many aspects of the earth. We call this the lunar cycle. Women are aligned to this cycle with their bodies and their moods, as are the oceans. When aspects of the world relate to divine feminine, nocturnal energies, or the aspects of earth regulated by the moon, this energy will be helpful in balancing these aspects.

Use: Invoke the energy using the regular process, and set the intention of which aspect of the moon needs balancing on earth. It could be that sleep cycles of humanity need to be balanced, as an example. Set the intention and say, "For the highest good of humanity and the earth." Allow the balancing to occur.

Example: Many of the hormones of women are currently out of balance due to a multitude of reasons that we will not get into. We could create an invocation such as: " **Menekryon, Menekryon, Menekryon**, realign the cycles and hormones of the divine feminine on earth to the natural cycles in alignment with the moon, in the highest good of women." Once we have created it, we will allow and simply watch as this evolves. These changes could occur in ways that women change the habits globally leading to the imbalances.

20. ASTERKRYON

Star Energy: This energy is related to the guidance of the stars. Much of our earth life is affected by the stars, albeit we have forgotten in modern times. There are many different beliefs and ancient texts about how the stars affect our daily lives. The Egyptians used astronomy for measurement and the creation of the pyramids. Humans throughout history have used the stars as a guidance system as well as a measurement tool. Scientists have many theories on how advanced the technology was in ancient times. My meditations and visions indicate that the technology was advanced and has been lost, as we forgot our origins and became covered in a veil. We are now at a point in time in which the veils are slowly being lifted, and humanity is once again connected to the stars and able to connect to the higher levels of awareness and consciousness.

Use: Use this energy to connect to the stars and bring in the wisdom and the powerful energy available. This energy is best utilized by receiving guidance through visions and meditations. The guidance and meditations provide the answers based on questions that are asked. Ask the question, invoke the energy, and allow the energy of the stars to guide you, similar to the way the ancients used to follow the stars.

21. AETHERKRYON

Ethers - The ethers are all which surrounds us. It is the air we breathe. From a scientific perspective it an oxygen atom connected to two alkyl or aryl groups. Our ethers can become out of balance and require balancing. There are many situations that could cause this, mostly human creations that no longer serve us. When the air we breathe is out of balance or unhealthy to breathe, this energy will balance it.

Use: Use this energy for any reason that the air is not in alignment with the highest good of humanity or earth. Invoke the energy using the invocation and set the intention of the part of the air that requires balancing. Place a platinum dome over the area that is being balanced with the mind's eye and imagine the murky unhealthy air being transformed into healthy, balanced air.

Example: In a densely populated city, it may sometimes become hard to breathe when there are few trees; this energy could be used to improve the air quality of the city. When it manifests it may be found that the city plants more trees, increases public transportation or there could be a big rain that clears the air.

22. GAMAKRYON

This is a ray of energy that emits large amounts of light energy. The **Gammakryon** energy is one of the strongest and most potent forms of energy available, that is in the form of a fine point, unlike the other energies, which cover large spaces or are all-encompassing in an aura or an area of the earth, This energy may be directed to small and very specific locations similar to a laser. The direction can be as fine as a small needle. The thickness of the energy may vary dependent upon the intention set by the healer. In Western medicine Gamma Rays are used to cure cancer and other diseases with light technology. We will use the "energetic, third eye" version, and not in exactly the same manner as the Western medical technology.

Examples of Use: The energy may be utilized for demarcation of boundaries between areas, and healing of the physical body. It is used in small spaces within the body for clearing out diseased areas where a pointed or fine ray is needed. This energy is generally intended to be used on living plant life, animals, or humans.

Use: Use the standard invocation process, set the intention, and direct the energy using the mind to the area or space where the energy is desired. For instance, if drawing a circle, use the mind's eye to direct the energy in a circle in the desired space.

Example: If the kidneys of a client are overworked, under severe stress and adrenal fatigue, the practitioner could use the mind's eye to direct the ray to the kidneys. The practitioner would then visualize the dark area where the excess stress resides and invoke the energy by saying: "**Gamakryon, Gamakryon, Gamakryon** clear stress and strengthen the kidneys to return them to full energetic functioning by filling them with the divine light of the **Gamakryon** energy." Finally, Imagine the kidneys filling with the **Gamakryon** light energy and healing.

Safety: This energy is not intended to replace any modern medical procedures or be used as a cure for anything. People with severe, chronic and life threatening conditions should continue to receive modern medical treatments. This energy may be used as a supplement to expedite or complement their medical treatments. This energy must be only directed to areas where the energy is truly needed or desired by someone who has the capability to direct energy. Always ask for the highest good through God for person who is receiving the healing. We must respect the divine plan for the person receiving the healing.

23. OMEGAKRYON

Ending: This energy is used to complete cycles or put an end to that which has already served it's purpose, and no longer serves us. There are many creations on earth now. Some of them serve our highest good, and some could be recreated in an improved way that serves the higher good for humanity or earth in the higher dimensions. This energy is best used for ending what no longer serves humanity or the earth at this time. Typically, it is best to use it with **Alphakryon**, as when a cycle ends, a new cycle begins. In order to have an ending, there must be a new beginning. It is best used by those light-workers who have practice clearing earthly issues and co-creating new ones.

Use: Invoke the energy and set the intention for that which no longer serves us. Be very specific in the intention. An entire system or process does not need to end because one aspect of it no longer serves us. Identify the area or portion that no longer serves us, and set that as the intention. Immediately set the intention for the creation or starting of the replacement process or system using **Alphakyron**. Refer to the first energy in this section for further explanation as these two energies are often paired.

Cautions: Ensure that when the intention is set, you are not creating havoc or disruption of systems. Avoid using this energy to create situations that would cause undue hardship on earth or humanity. Always ask for the highest good, one with God. There is always a break pedal with all of the energies, so changes will only come into fruition if manifested from the high vibration of love and the highest good.

Example if the mail system we use is very slow, there is no reason to do away with the whole system. Set the intention to end the portions of the systems that are causing the slow down. An intention for this invocation could be: "**Omegakryon** all processes within the mail system that block the highest efficiency, **Alphakryon** new processes that allow mail to flow freely at the highest efficiency in the highest good for all involved and in alignment with God."

Example; if the world is using excessive amounts of disposable plastic that fill landfills and pollute oceans, the invocation could go:

"**Omegkryon** excessive use of disposable plastics, **Alphakryon** to reduce, re-use and recycle plastic products or the highest good of the planet." One could also activate **Pimikryon** with this activation to cleanse the environment.

24: TWIN RAYS

These two rays are used for healing from the perspective of balancing the divine feminine and masculine.

PLATINUM PINK RAY

The platinum ray looks exactly as it sounds, like a ray of platinum with an undertone of pink colored energy. The ray is activated using the healers third eye or mind's eye. Use this ray to activate a specific site on earth with the divine feminine energy or within a human body. When invoked it will bring in the divine feminine energy to an area for healing.

ELECTRIC BLUE RAY

The blue ray is an electric blue color that looks similar to the electric blue color of a vibrant ocean or the Mediterranean sky. This ray is also activated from the healer's third eye or mind's eye, and is representative of the divine masculine.

Purpose: The purpose of the Twin rays is for balancing the divine feminine and masculine. The earth and humanity have been going through a process of raising in vibration, and in order to do this the divine feminine and masculine must be perfectly balanced in humans as well as earth. Earlier in the book, we discussed the **Ankryon** energy for balancing the divine feminine and masculine, we also discussed that the location for this balancing occurs in the third chakra, the seat of the soul, also known as the solar plexus. The energy of **Ankryon** may be used in combination with the Twin Rays in order to balance the feminine and masculine within a human or earthly locations. In order for our bodies and earth to increase in vibration, it is imperative that these energies be balanced regularly.

It is quite noticeable that equality of women has been increasing exponentially over the past 100 years and more and more, and the lines of roles between the sexes have blurred. The earth is going through a balancing of these energy in her own chakra system simultaneously to the human shift. The progress is tremendous.

Many spiritually awakened humans on earth have been meeting what may be termed as twin flames. These twins are typically a male and female, although sometimes same sex, that share a soul signature and are drawn together for spiritual work with what feels like a magnet.

At the beginning of this era, the souls split into two in order to experience lessons in duality. We are now reaching a point in which the souls are ready to return to oneness and rebalance to become whole again. The twins may or may not have a romantic relationship. What is more important is the deep soul connection and vibration that they share. Some twins have multiple twin flames, and may connect with more than one at the soul level however, most have only one. When there is more than one, that means that the soul has divided into more than two bodies to increase the level of lessons in duality. These meetings are important to the growth and raising of vibration of earth and humanity as these relationships are balancing these energies simply by these twins working together to resolve differences in duality. Often times the twins will have a spiritual purpose or work to do here on earth. The rays may be used to assist with these relationships. The balancing may be done on one or both of the twin flames. The balancing will occur either way.

Invocation of the Rays:

Single Ray Invocation: Imagine with the Mind's Eye that the ray is coming down from the heavens, and like a light beam is directed at the person, place or thing where the balancing is to occur.

Places: Generally the rays will work within a specific single point or location, and radiate over a larger space, which could cover several meters or miles in diameter depending on the intention set by the healer.

> *Example: If the ray were to be initiated over the peak of a mountain, it would be directed through the apex of the mountain, and the energy of the ray would radiate through the entire mountain filling the space of the mountain with the energy.*

Person: When working with a person, imagine with the mind's eye that the ray is directed to the specific area of the aura or physical body where the work is being done.

> *Example: If the heart chakra is out of balance in regards to the divine feminine, the platinum pink ray would be directed toward this chakra for healing. The healer would visualize that the chakra is filled with the ray.*

Twin Ray Invocation: Imagine that the two rays of electric blue and platinum pink are intertwined in a double helix similar to that of a DNA strand.

- **Places:** Imagine with the mind's eye that the double helix of the twin energies is directed into the area that requires the two energies to be balanced.

- **Person:** Imagine with the mind's eye that the double helix of the twin energies is aligned with the spine of the patient, starting with the bottom of the helix at the base of the sacral or first chakra and goes up to a minimum of the crown or seventh chakra, as far up to the sixteenth chakra.

Invocation Words: While imagining the helix in the space or along the spine, the following invocation will be said:

"The divine feminine and divine masculine are perfectly balanced in harmony, peace, unity, oneness, prosperity in alignment with the highest Christ self and the divine plan ONE with God."

Once the invocation is complete, the balancing has occurred. This can be repeated over multiple sessions. Even with only one session, the effects will be profound.

Time: As we have mentioned throughout the book, the energies work within a non-linear time frame, so simply allow and accept the changes will occur according to divine timing.

ABOUT THE AUTHOR

Dr. Sara Florida L.Ac, PhD, is an integrative medicine practitioner in Texas. She specializes in mood and emotional disorders as well as digestive health. She focuses on how the various aspects of health—including mood, energy levels, and brain function—are related to the digestive function. Her treatments and therapies treat all these areas for whole-health healing. In addition to Oriental medicine, she uses yoga, meditation, and qigong therapy to help her patients with balance, injuries, pain, and mental emotional well-being. Her own twenty year journey of reading literature, studying and attending workshops have led to her current knowledge and expertise.

She is an intuitive empath and uses her natural gifts in her healing. She uses the twenty four energies advanced healing technology for interdimensional healing in her practice to release emotional blockages and disorders from all levels of the body. She does this by permission and when appropriate. Her doctoral studies are in Spiritual Healing from the University of Sedona where she is completing her dissertation. Her master's degree is in Oriental medicine, she is certified in functional medicine, as a yoga instructor in Ashtanga yoga, and has studies in qigong and tai qi. She has been relentlessly researching emotional health, digestive health, and yoga since the 1990s at conferences and through literature as part of her own healing journey.

REFERENCES

Cayce, Edgar. *The Power of Your Mind (Edgar Cayce Series Title)*. 2010

Cota-Robles, Patricia. *The Next Step…Re-Unification with the Presence of God Within Our Hearts*. 1989.

Cota-Robles, Patricia. *The Violet Flame: God's Gift to Humanity*. 2005.

Cross, John R. and Robert Charman. *Healing with the Chakra Energy System: Acupressure, Bodywork, and Reflexology for Total Health*. 2006.

Dale, Cyndi. *Advanced Chakra Healing*. 2005.

Dale, Cyndi. *The Subtle Body: An Encyclopedia of Your Energetic Anatomy*. 2009.

Hall, Judy. *The Art of Psychic Protection*. 2011.

Hofstadter, Douglas R. and Daniel C. Dennett. *The Mind's I: Fantasies and Reflections on Self & Soul*. 2001

McLaren, Karla. *Your Aura & Your Chakras: The Owner's Manual*. 1998.

Miller, David K. *New Spiritual Technology for the Fifth-Dimensional Earth: Arcturian Teachings from the Sacred Triangle*. 2009.

Sankey, Mikio. *Esoteric Acupuncture: Gateway to Expanded Healing, Vol. 1*. 1999.

Skinner, Stephen. *Sacred Geometry: Deciphering the Code*. 2009

Tyberonn, James. *The Alchemy of Ascension*. 2010.

Wetzel, Lois J. *Akashic Records: Case Studies of Past Lives*. 2011.

Weissman, Dr. Darren R. *Awakening to the Secret Code of Your Mind: Your Mind's Journey to Inner Peace*. 2010.

Wojton, Djuna. *Karmic Healing: Clearing Past-Life Blocks to Present-Day Love, Health, and Happiness*. 2014.

I offer this book to healers and light workers as a gift of healing from the higher angelic realms, light beings and God. May this book bring about peace, love, light, unity, oneness and prosperity in alignment with the highest divine purpose of healing humanity and earth.

~Love Sara

Made in the USA
Monee, IL
15 December 2019